MW00891581

WHEN I GO LOW

Written By Ginger Vieira
Illustrated By Mike Lawson

Text copyright © 2020 by Ginger Vieira
Illustrations copyright © 2020 by Mike Lawson
All rights reserved, including the right of reproduction in whole or in part in any form.
For more information visit MrMikeLawson.com & GingerVieira.com

Dedicated to our friends in the diabetes community who help us each learn about our lows, our highs, and everything in between.

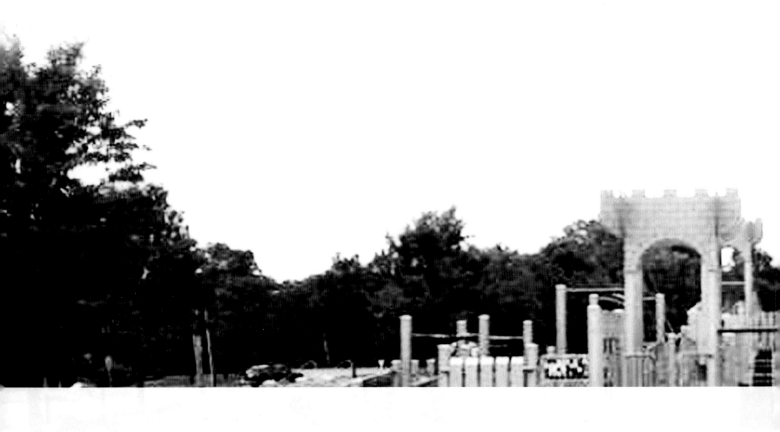

Jax the Cat has type 1 diabetes.
Sometimes he wishes he didn't.

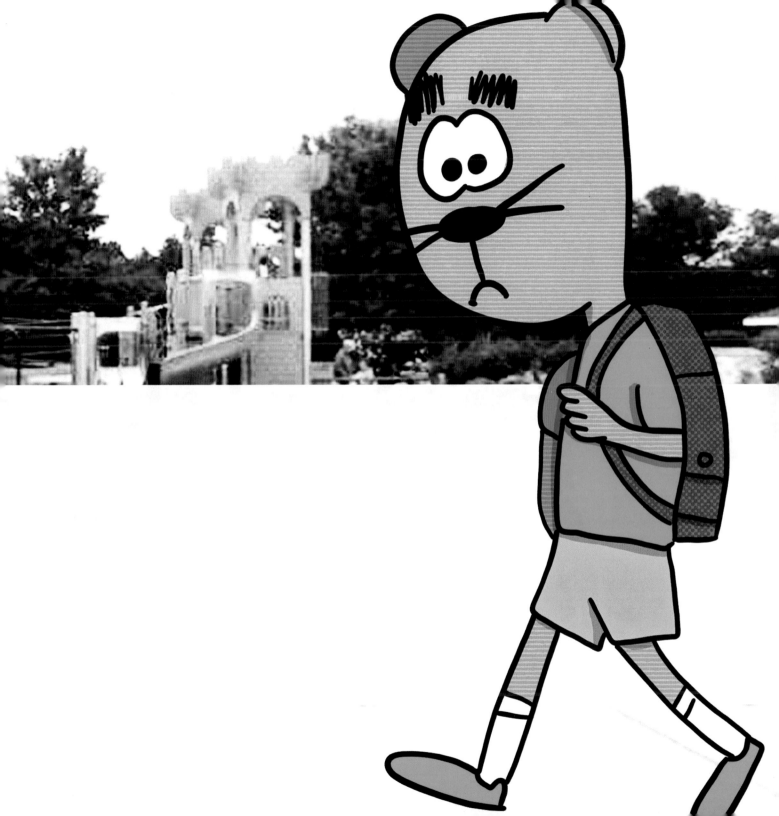

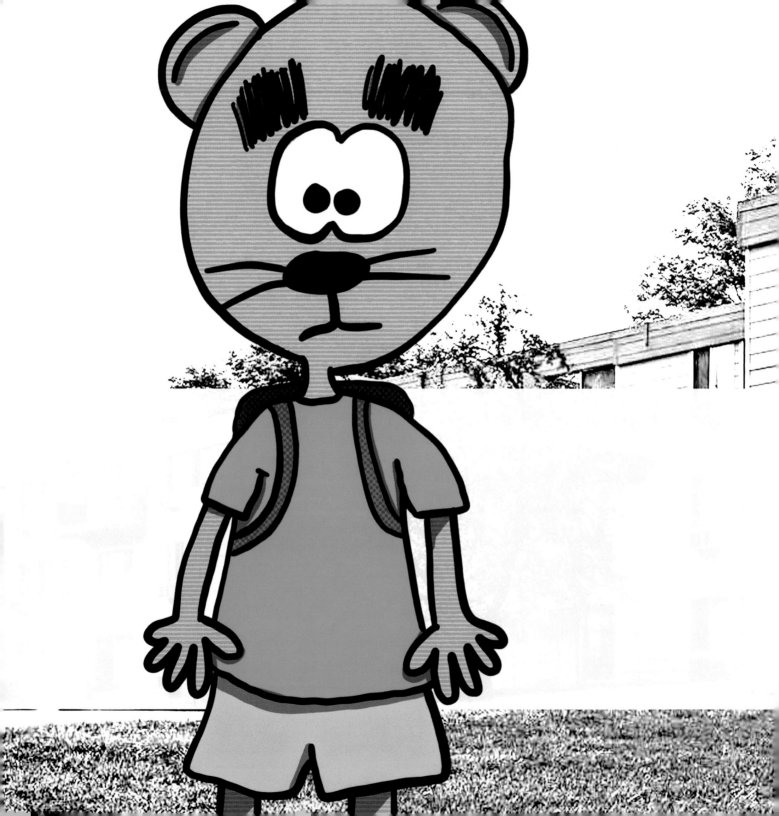

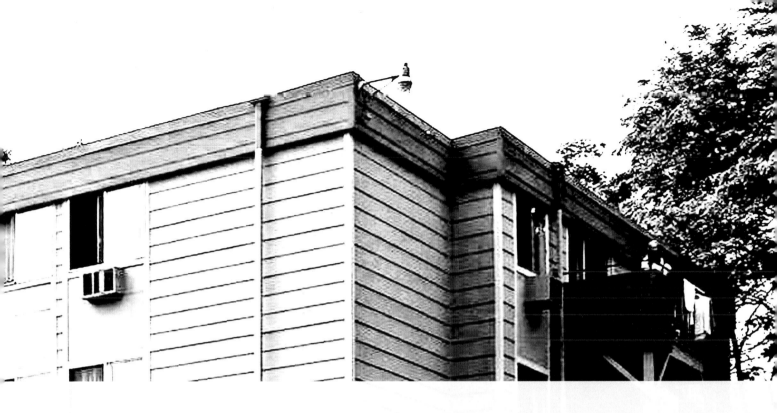

"I feel like the only kid in town with diabetes," says Jax.

"Besides all the finger pokes and taking my insulin, what bothers me the most is when I go low."

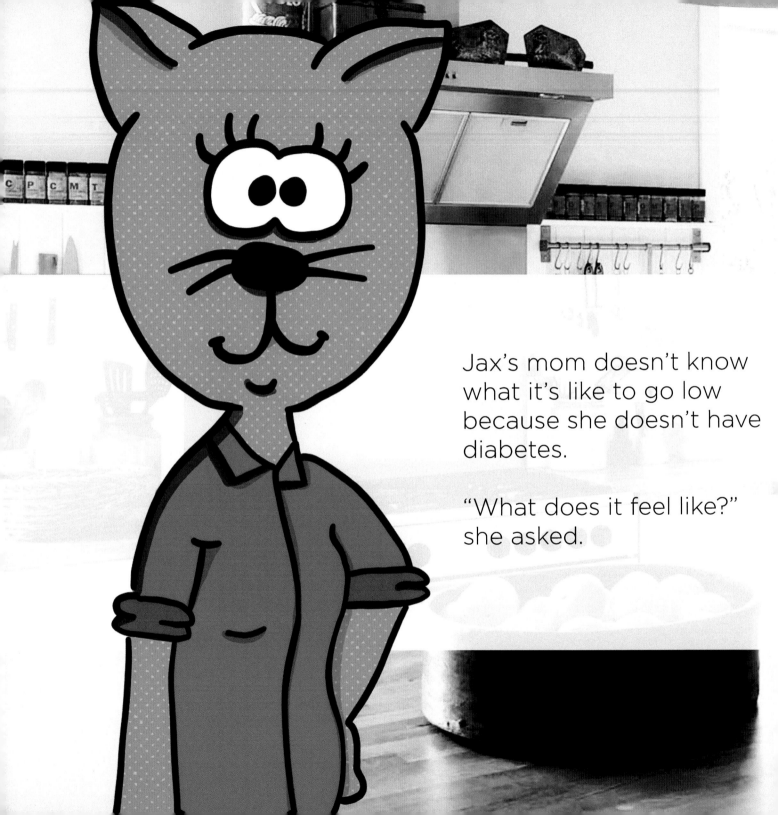

Jax's mom doesn't know what it's like to go low because she doesn't have diabetes.

"What does it feel like?" she asked.

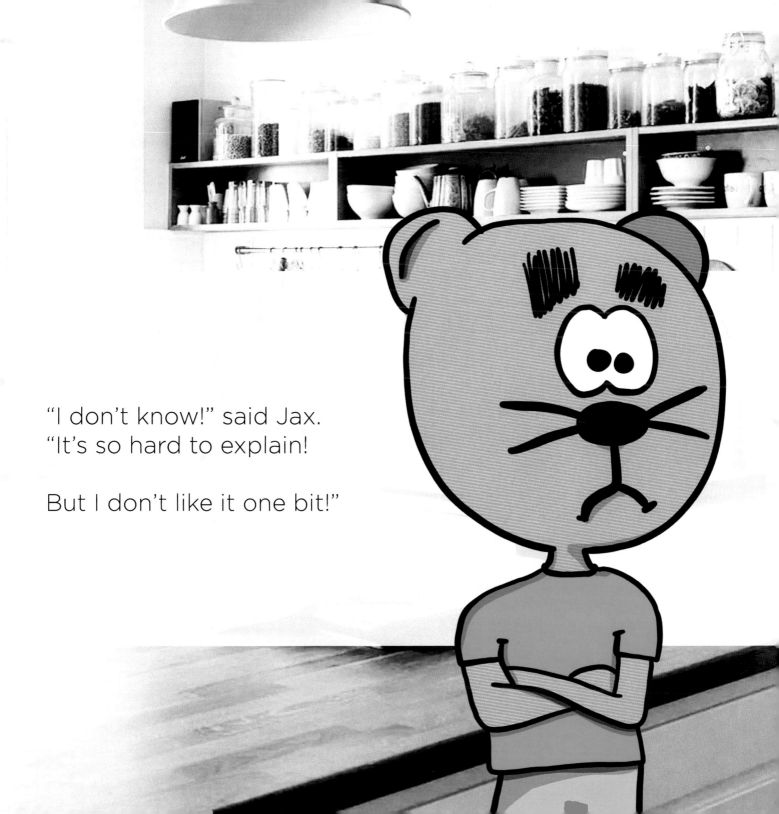

"I don't know!" said Jax.
"It's so hard to explain!

But I don't like it one bit!"

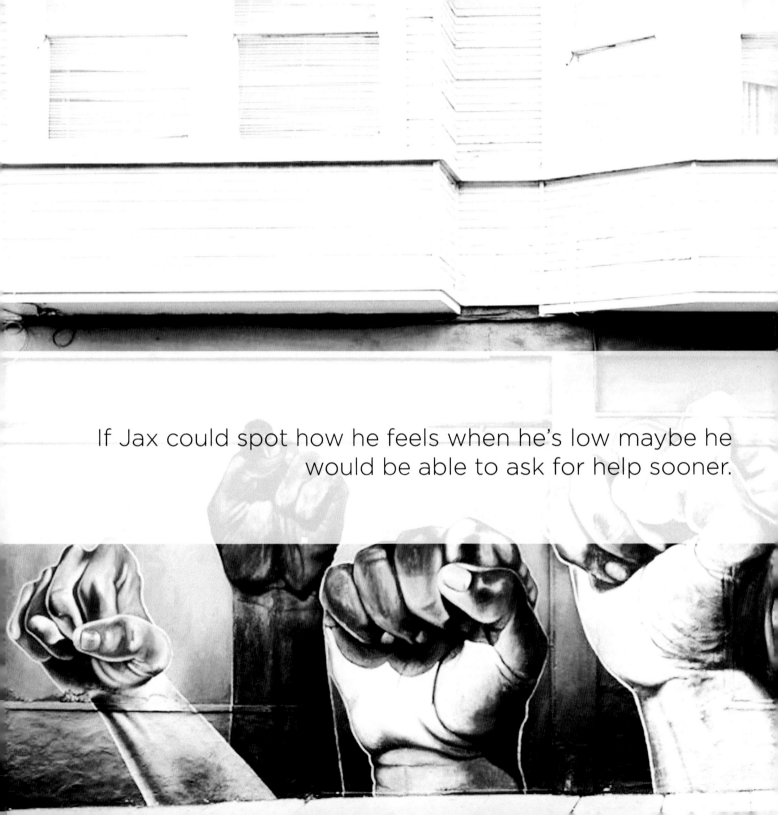

If Jax could spot how he feels when he's low maybe he would be able to ask for help sooner.

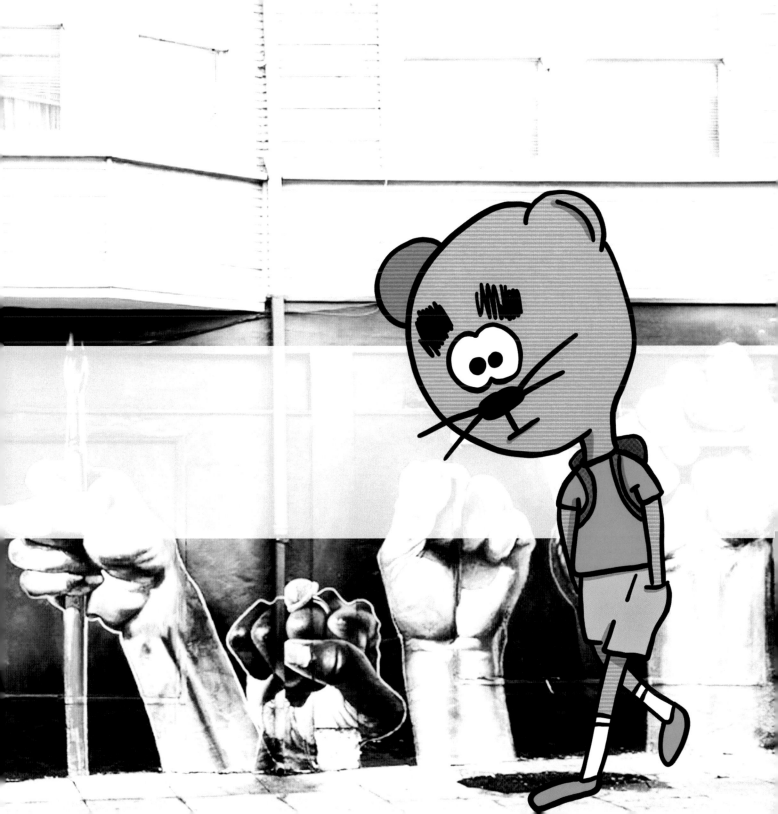

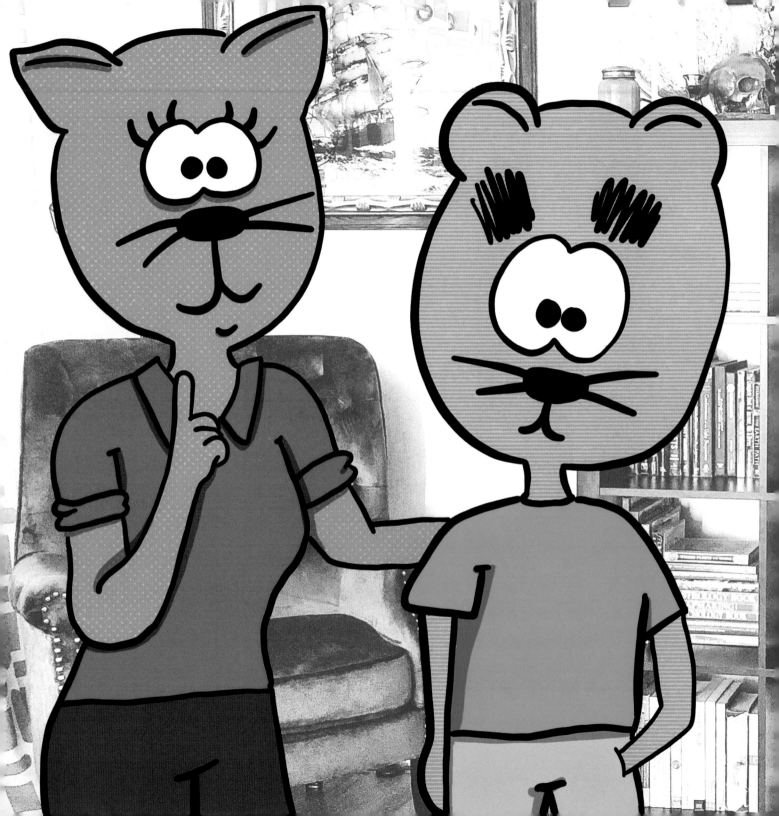

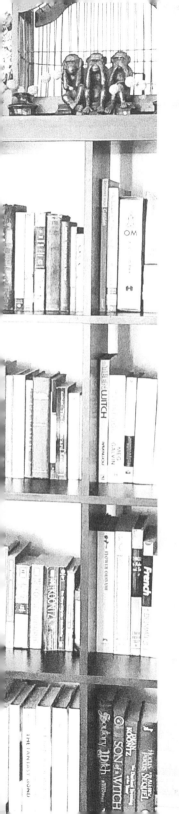
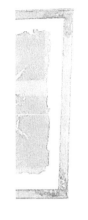

"You know," said Mom, "you're not the only kid with diabetes."

"I'm not?" said Jax. He couldn't believe it! Other kids just like him have to deal with finger pokes and taking their insulin, too? And counting carbs? And planning everything around diabetes all the time?

"I'm gonna find these other kids!" said Jax.

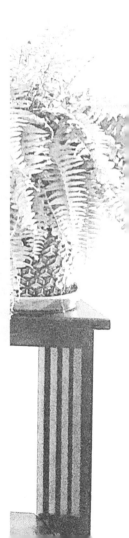

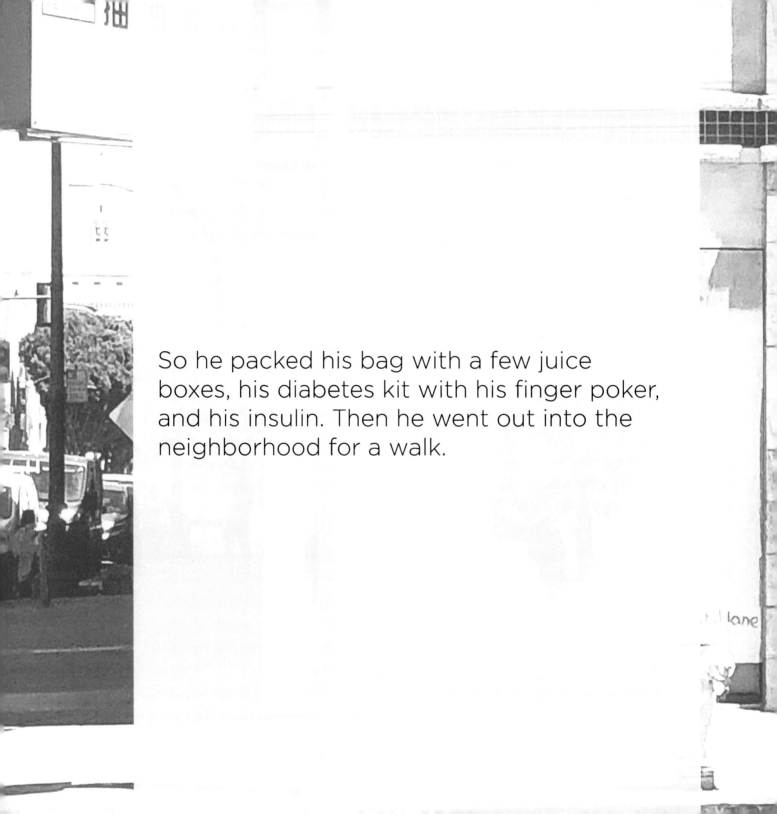

So he packed his bag with a few juice boxes, his diabetes kit with his finger poker, and his insulin. Then he went out into the neighborhood for a walk.

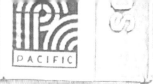
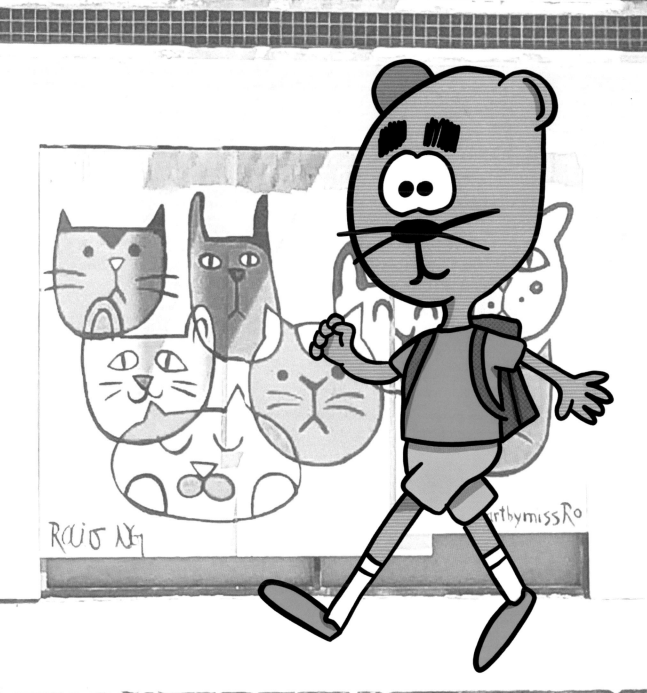

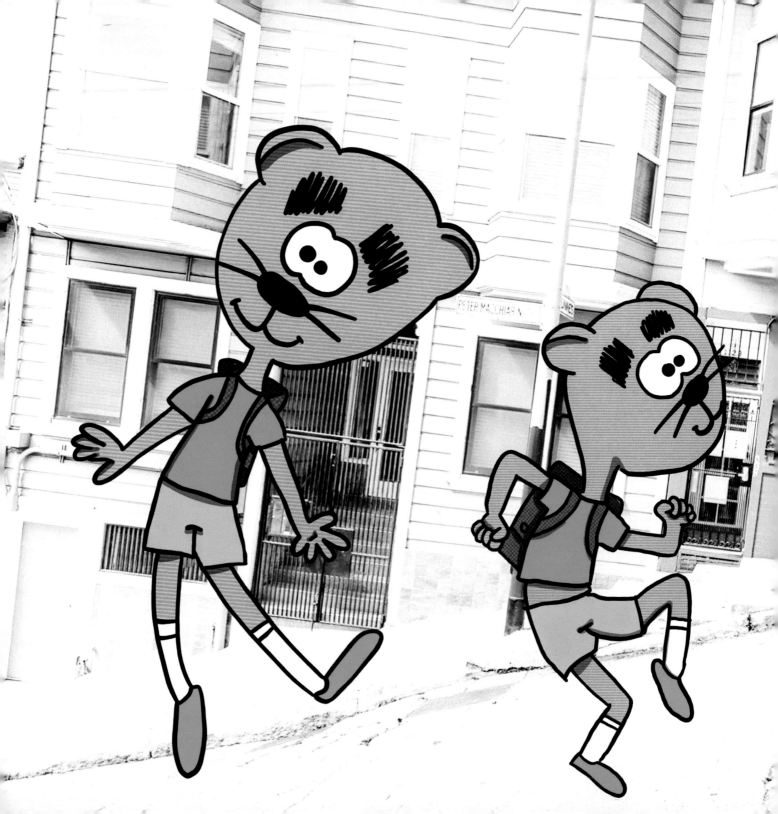

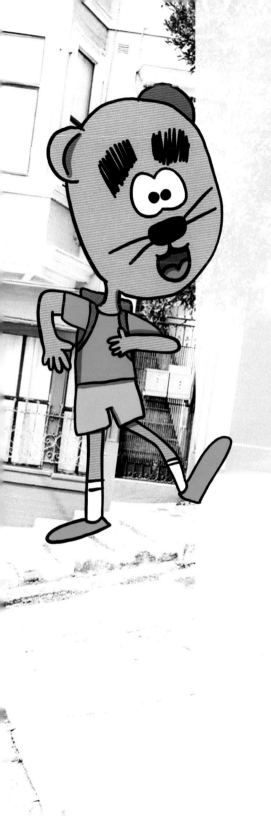

When I go low
I feel so, so, so
Wibbily, wobbily
Flibbily, flobbily

When I go low
That's how I know
It's time to eat
My special treat

I eat my treat
To get back on my feet
Feeling ready to play
For the rest of the day!

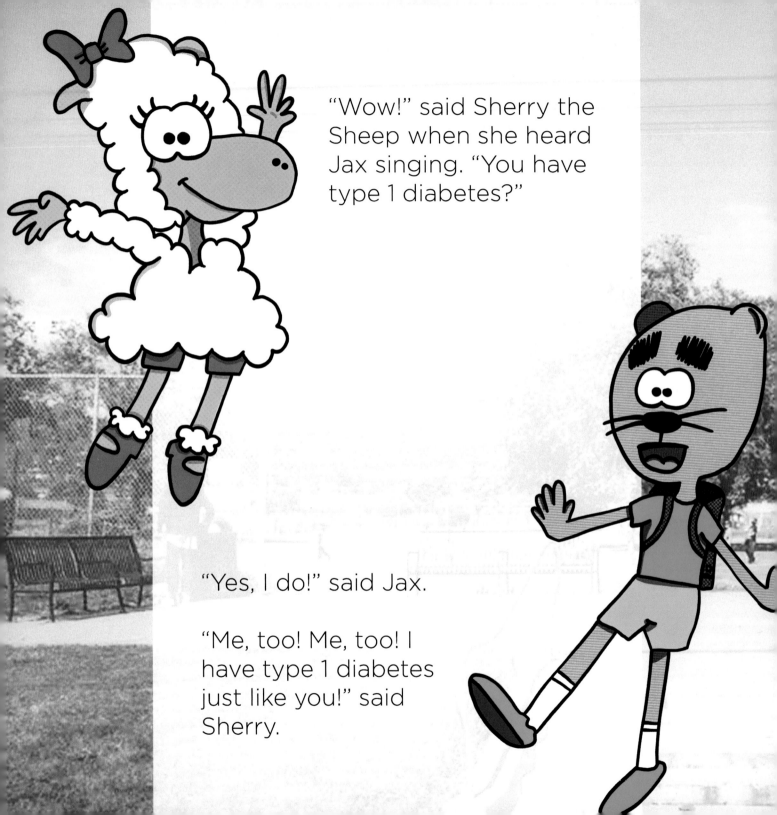

"Wow!" said Sherry the Sheep when she heard Jax singing. "You have type 1 diabetes?"

"Yes, I do!" said Jax.

"Me, too! Me, too! I have type 1 diabetes just like you!" said Sherry.

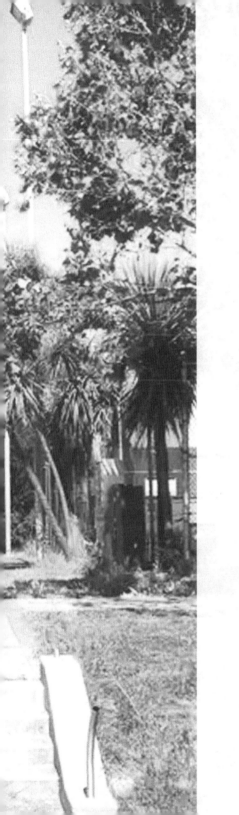

"Wow! And...do you go low sometimes, too?"

"I do! I do! I do!" said Sherry. "When I go low, I feel shaky, shaky, shaky!"

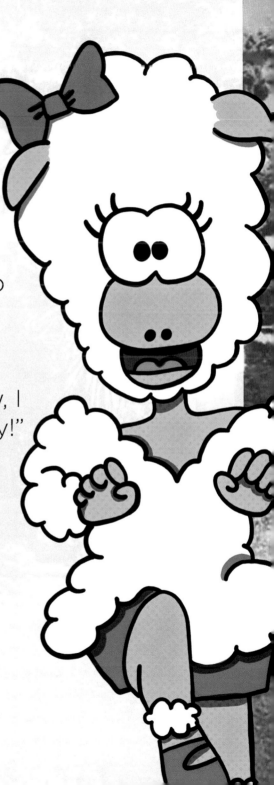

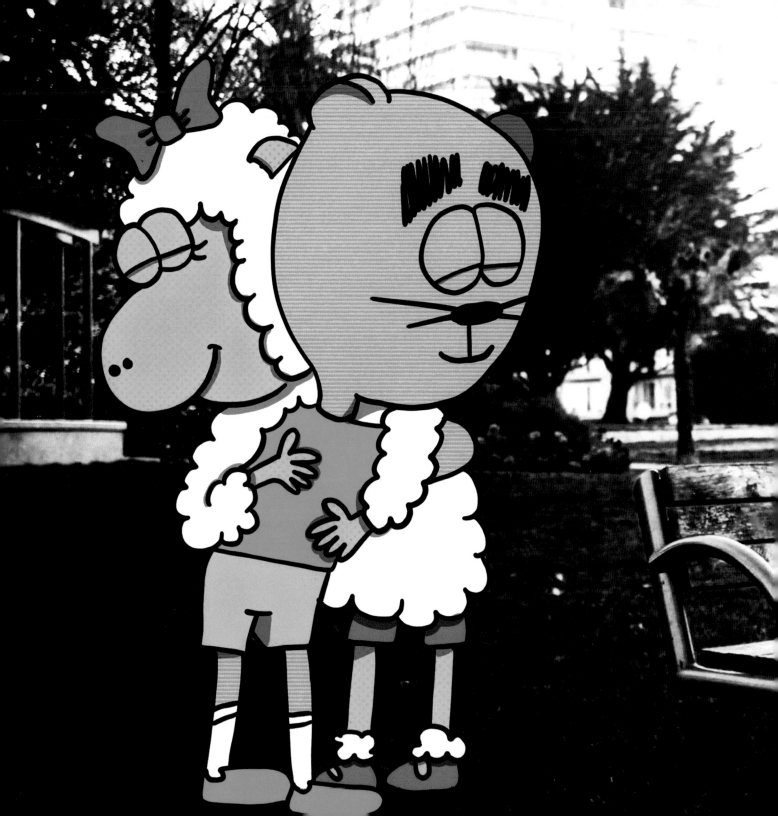

Jax said, "You know, when I go low, I feel shaky, shaky, shaky, too!"

Jax the Cat gave Sherry the Sheep a big, big hug because they both know just how brave they have to be to deal with diabetes every single day.

Then Jax continued on his walking journey to find other kids in town.

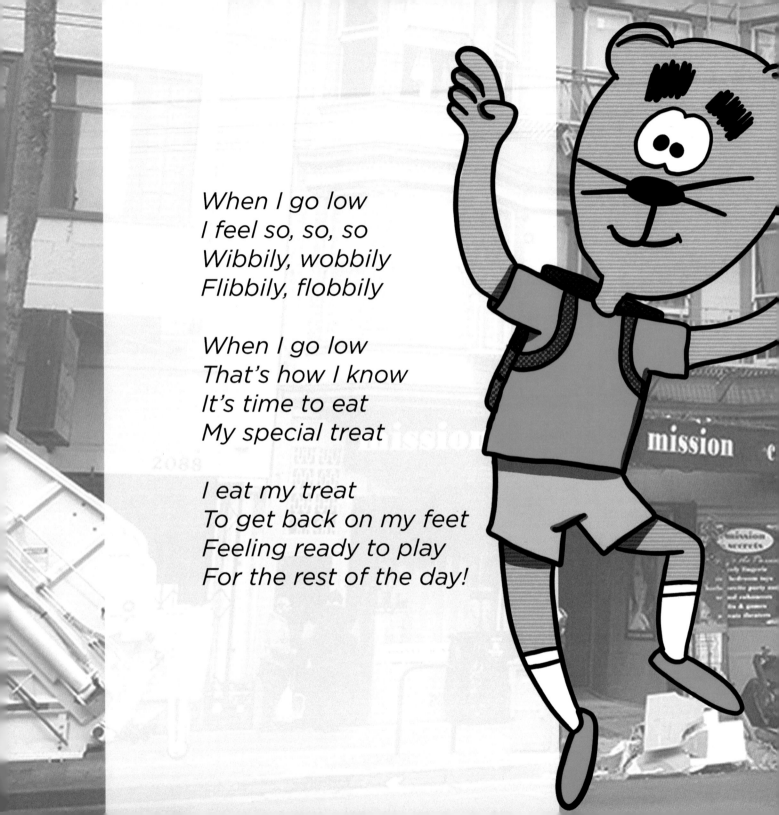

When I go low
I feel so, so, so
Wibbily, wobbily
Flibbily, flobbily

When I go low
That's how I know
It's time to eat
My special treat

I eat my treat
To get back on my feet
Feeling ready to play
For the rest of the day!

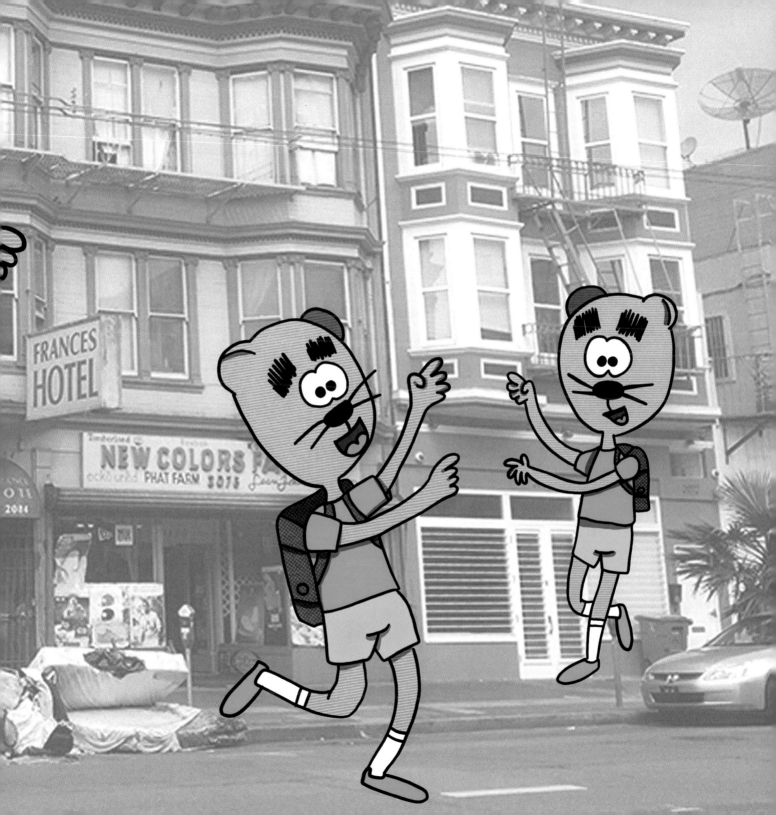

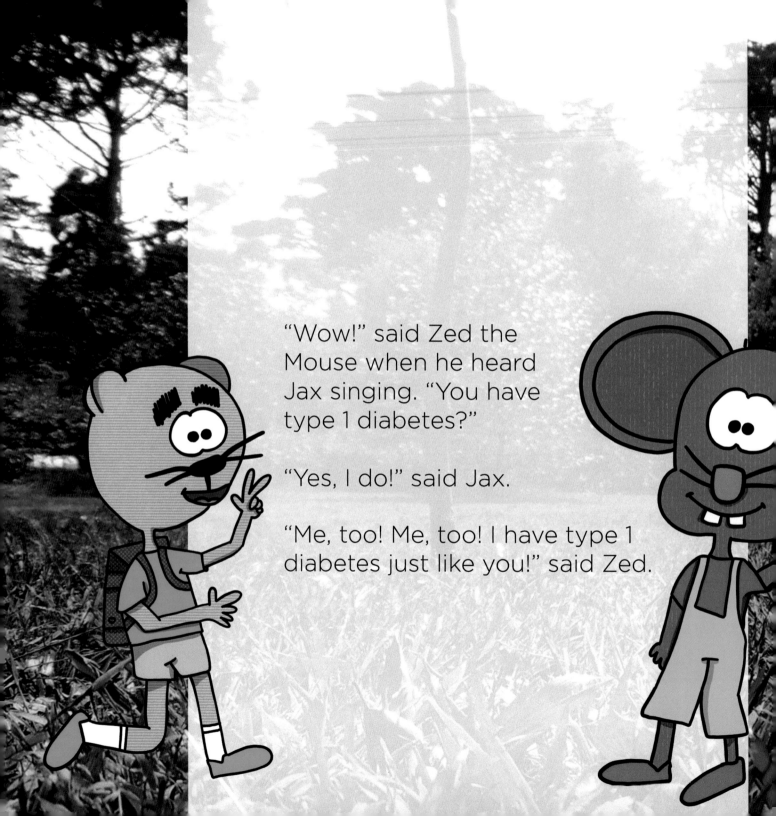

"Wow!" said Zed the Mouse when he heard Jax singing. "You have type 1 diabetes?"

"Yes, I do!" said Jax.

"Me, too! Me, too! I have type 1 diabetes just like you!" said Zed.

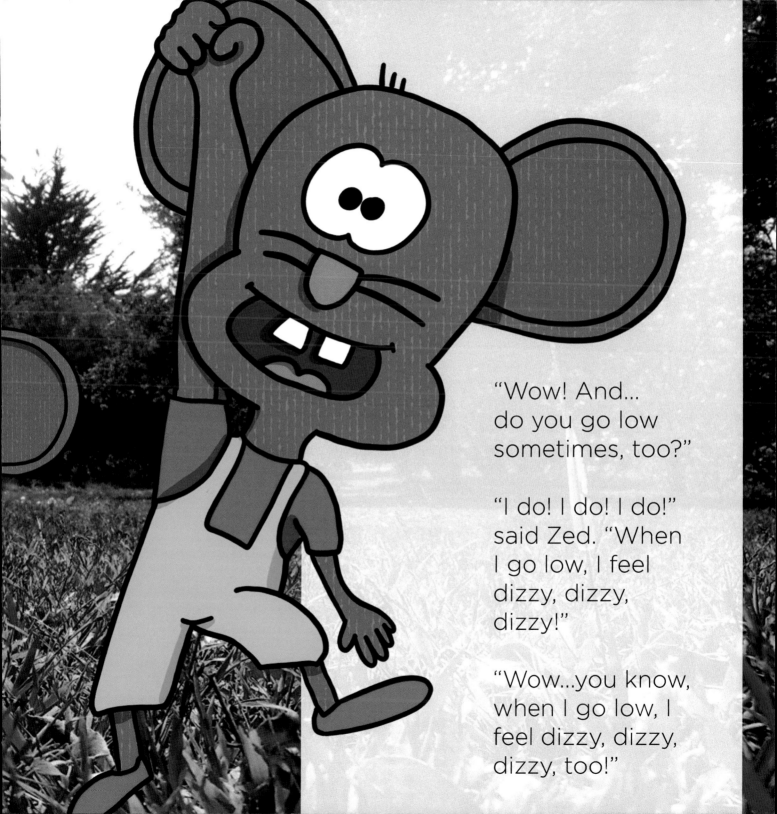

"Wow! And...
do you go low
sometimes, too?"

"I do! I do! I do!"
said Zed. "When
I go low, I feel
dizzy, dizzy,
dizzy!"

"Wow...you know,
when I go low, I
feel dizzy, dizzy,
dizzy, too!"

Jax the Cat gave Zed the Mouse a big, big hug because they both know just how brave they have to be to deal with diabetes every single day.

Then Jax continued on his walking journey to find other kids in town with diabetes.

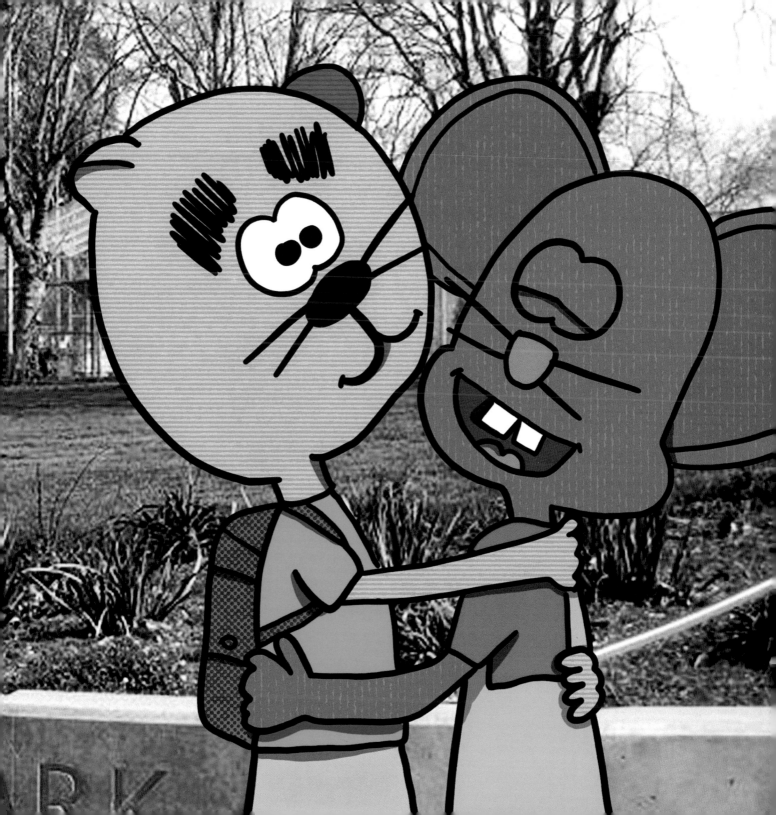

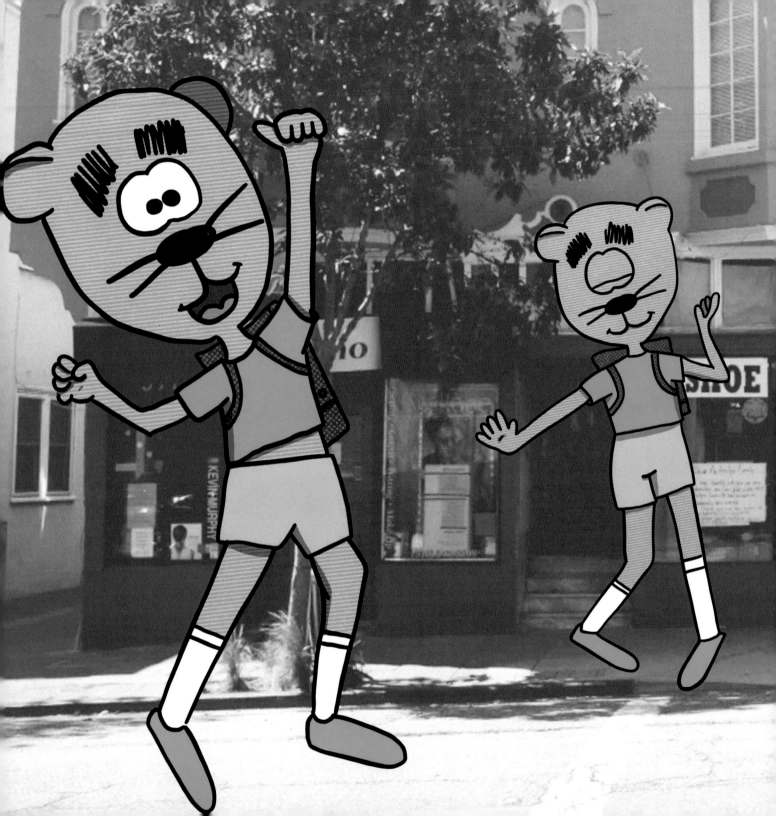

When I go low
I feel so, so, so
Wibbily, wobbily
Flibbily, flobbily

When I go low
That's how I know
It's time to eat
My special treat

I eat my treat
To get back on my feet
Feeling ready to play
For the rest of the day!

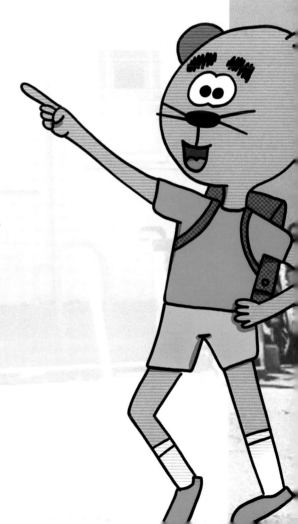

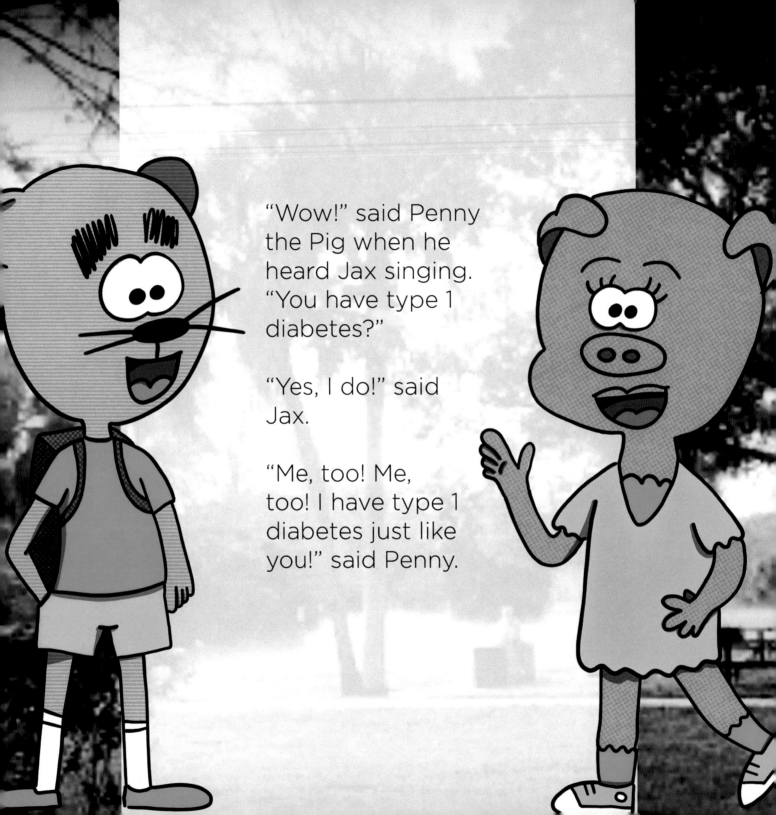

"Wow!" said Penny the Pig when he heard Jax singing. "You have type 1 diabetes?"

"Yes, I do!" said Jax.

"Me, too! Me, too! I have type 1 diabetes just like you!" said Penny.

"Wow! And... do you go low sometimes, too?"

"I do! I do! I do!" said Penny. "When I go low, I feel mad, mad, mad!"

"Wow...you know, when I go low, I feel mad, mad, mad, too!"

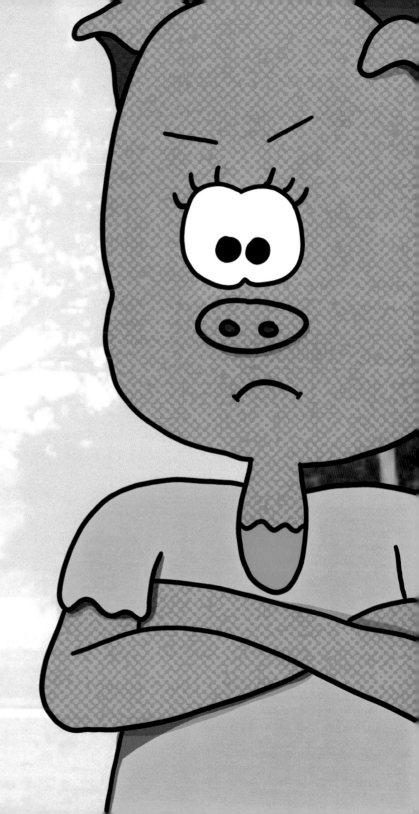

Jax the Cat gave Penny the Pig a big, big hug because they both know just how brave they have to be to deal with diabetes every single day.

Then Jax continued on his walking journey to find other kids in town.

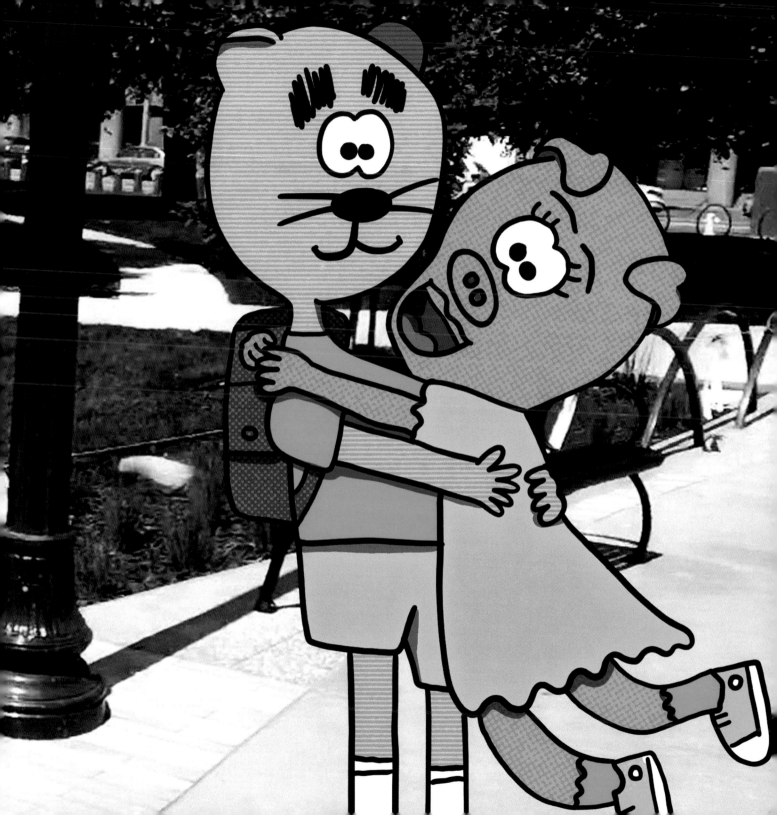

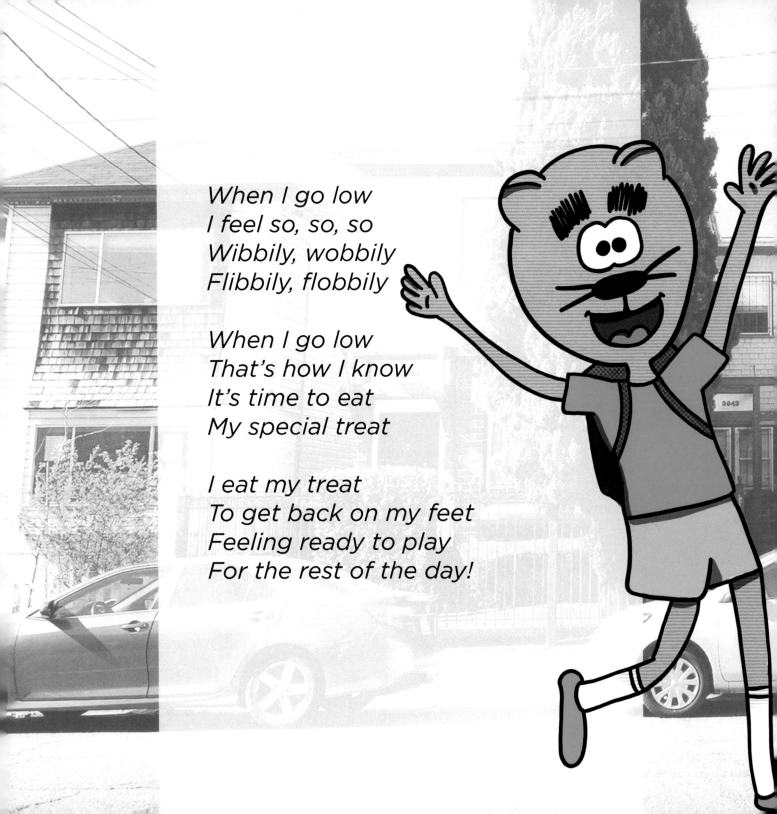

When I go low
I feel so, so, so
Wibbily, wobbily
Flibbily, flobbily

When I go low
That's how I know
It's time to eat
My special treat

I eat my treat
To get back on my feet
Feeling ready to play
For the rest of the day!

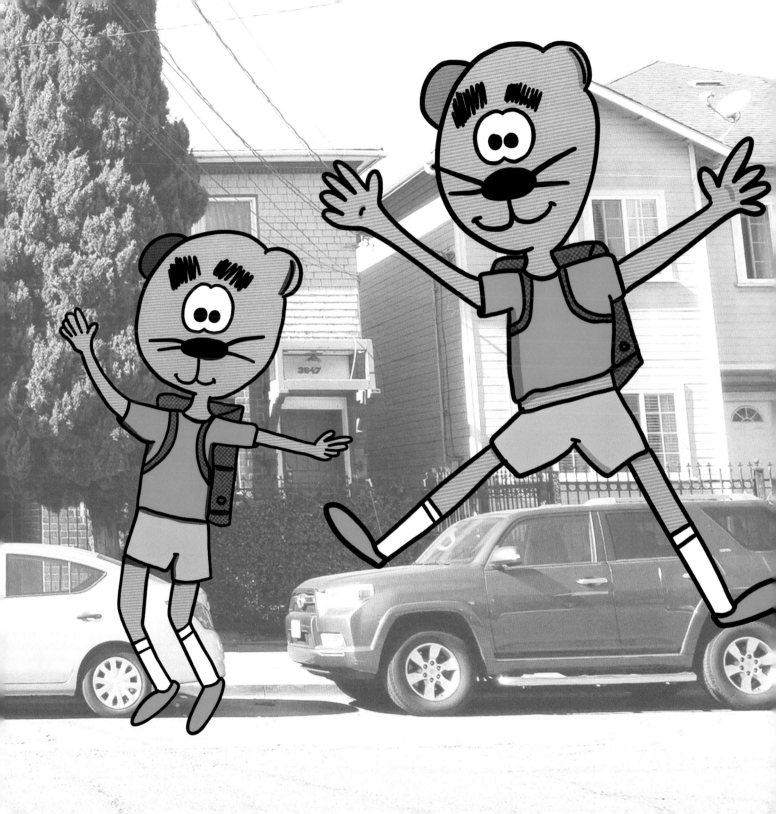

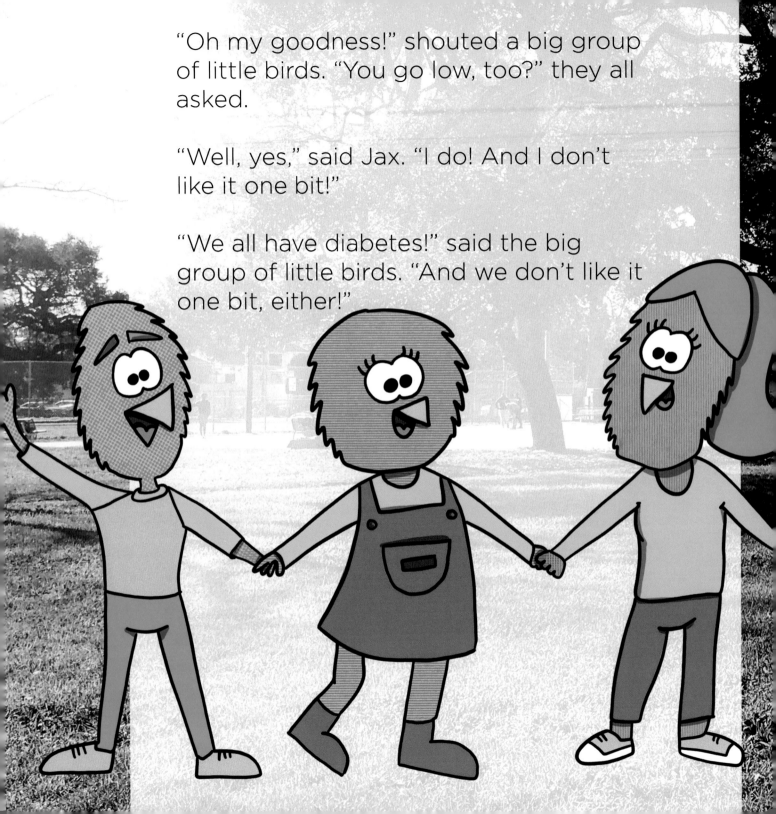

"Oh my goodness!" shouted a big group of little birds. "You go low, too?" they all asked.

"Well, yes," said Jax. "I do! And I don't like it one bit!"

"We all have diabetes!" said the big group of little birds. "And we don't like it one bit, either!"

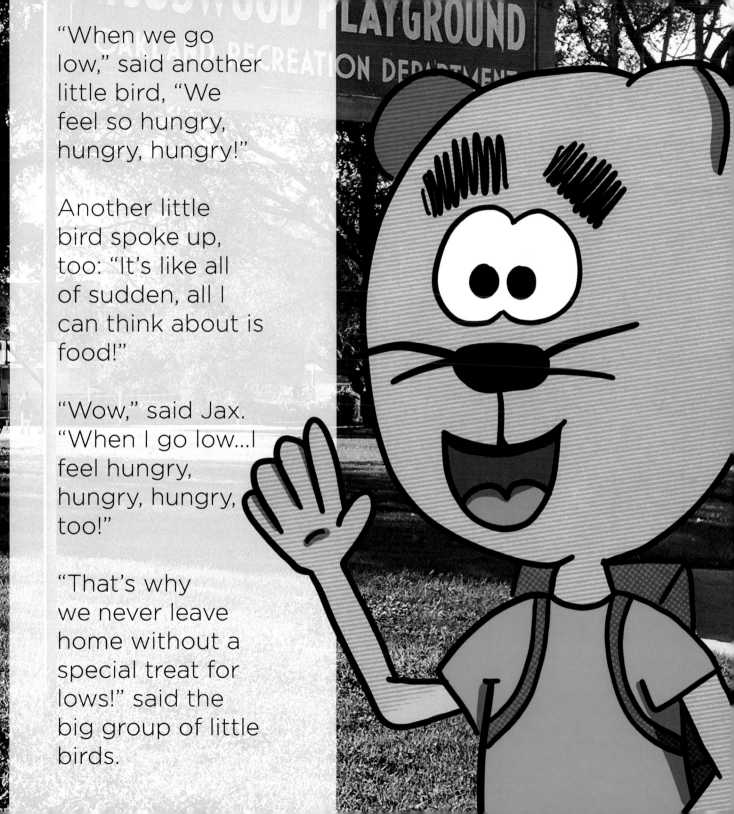

"When we go low," said another little bird, "We feel so hungry, hungry, hungry!"

Another little bird spoke up, too: "It's like all of sudden, all I can think about is food!"

"Wow," said Jax. "When I go low...I feel hungry, hungry, hungry, too!"

"That's why we never leave home without a special treat for lows!" said the big group of little birds.

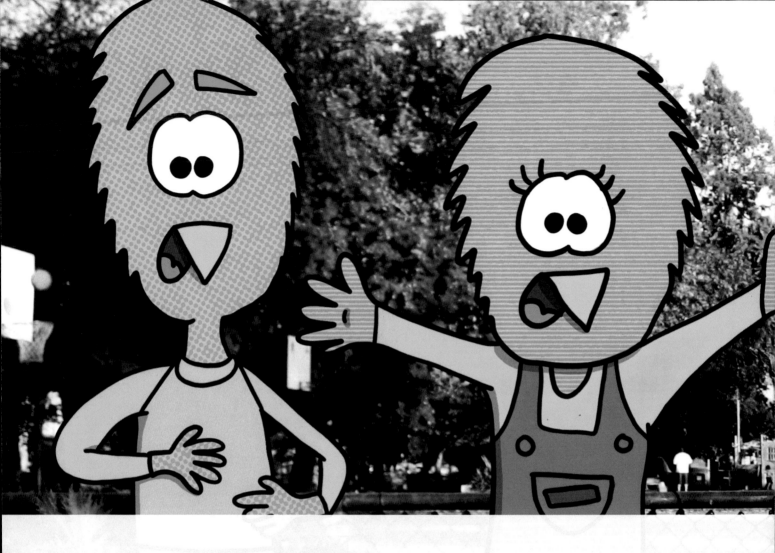

"And we know there are so many other kids in town who have diabetes like you and me," said the big group of little birds.

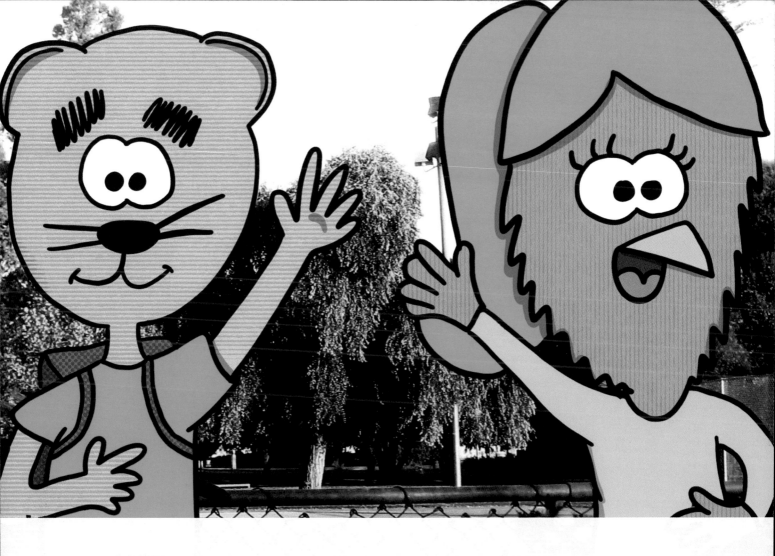

"We just have to be brave!" said Jax.

"We do! We do! We do!" said the big group of little birds.

Jax quickly ran home to tell Mom Cat about his adventure.

"Mom! I met so many other kids in town who have type 1 diabetes just like me!"

But then, after all of that walking, Jax realized he was starting to feel...shaky, and dizzy, and mad, and hungry!

"Oh my goodness!" said Jax. "I'm feeling all of the things my new friends with diabetes feel when they go low!"

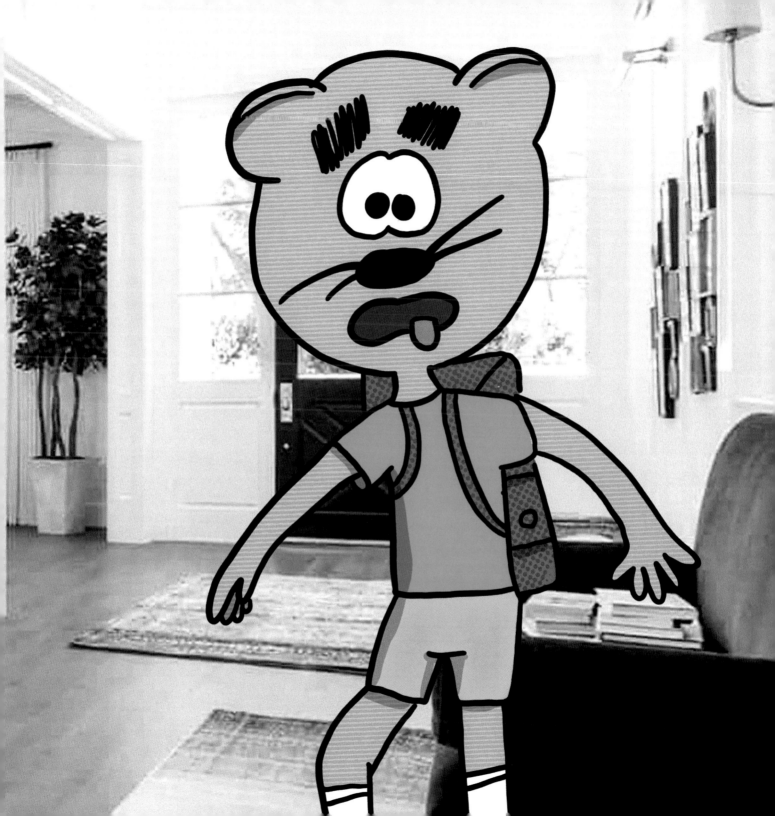

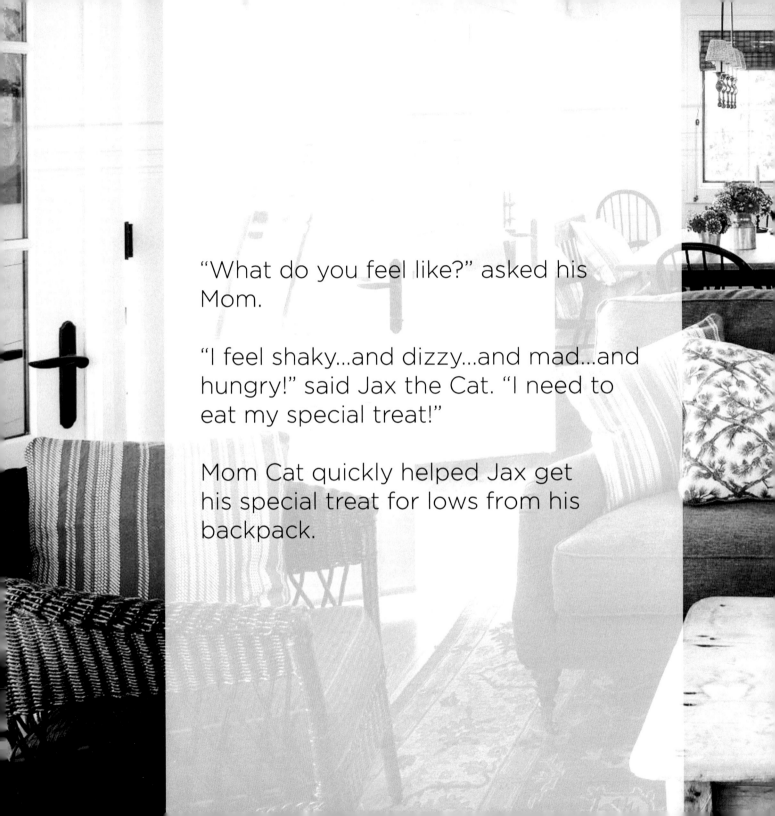

"What do you feel like?" asked his Mom.

"I feel shaky...and dizzy...and mad...and hungry!" said Jax the Cat. "I need to eat my special treat!"

Mom Cat quickly helped Jax get his special treat for lows from his backpack.

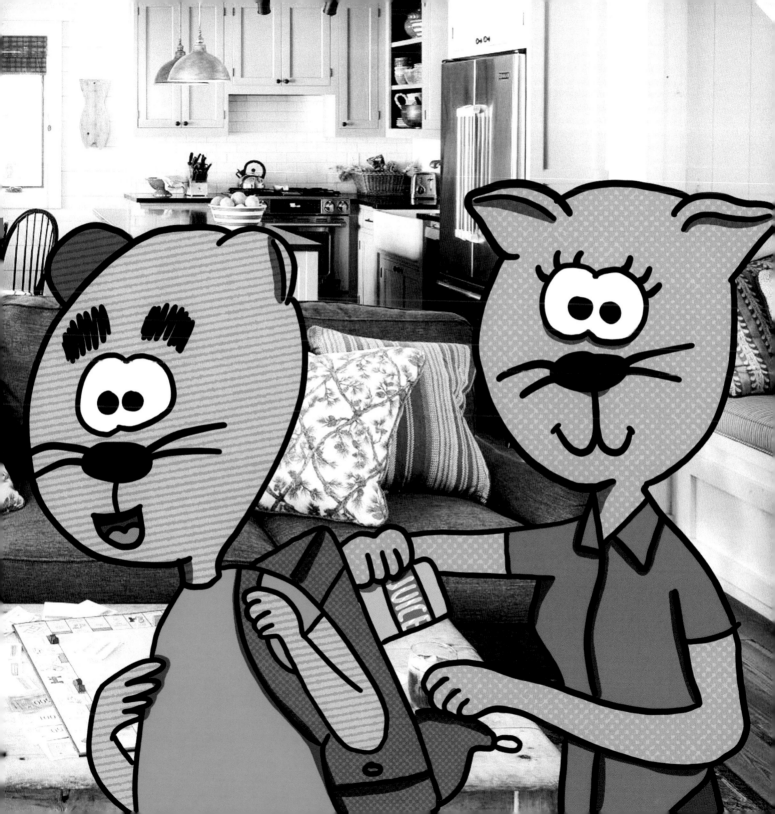

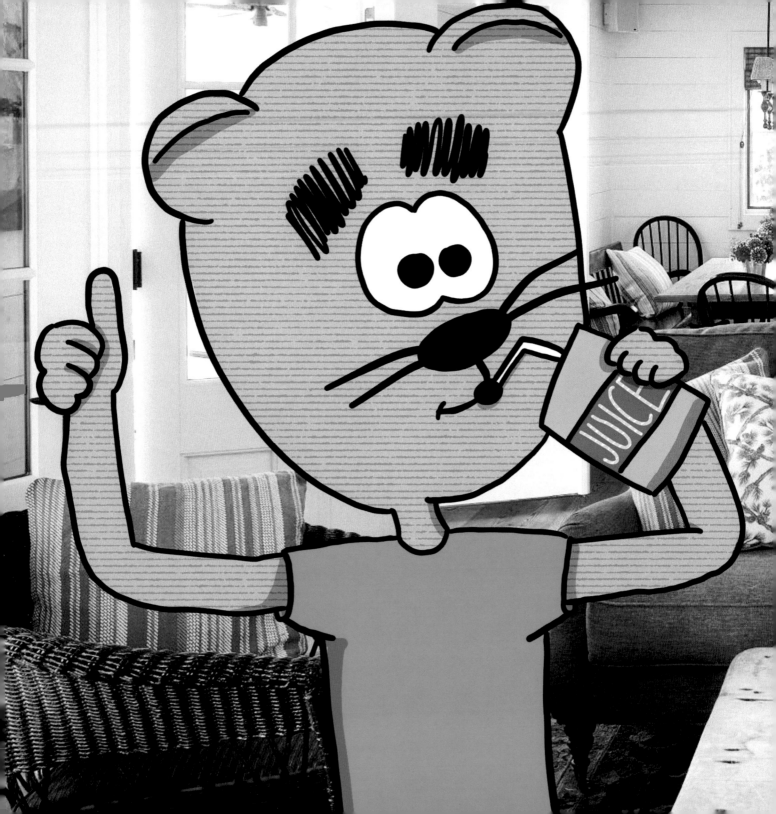

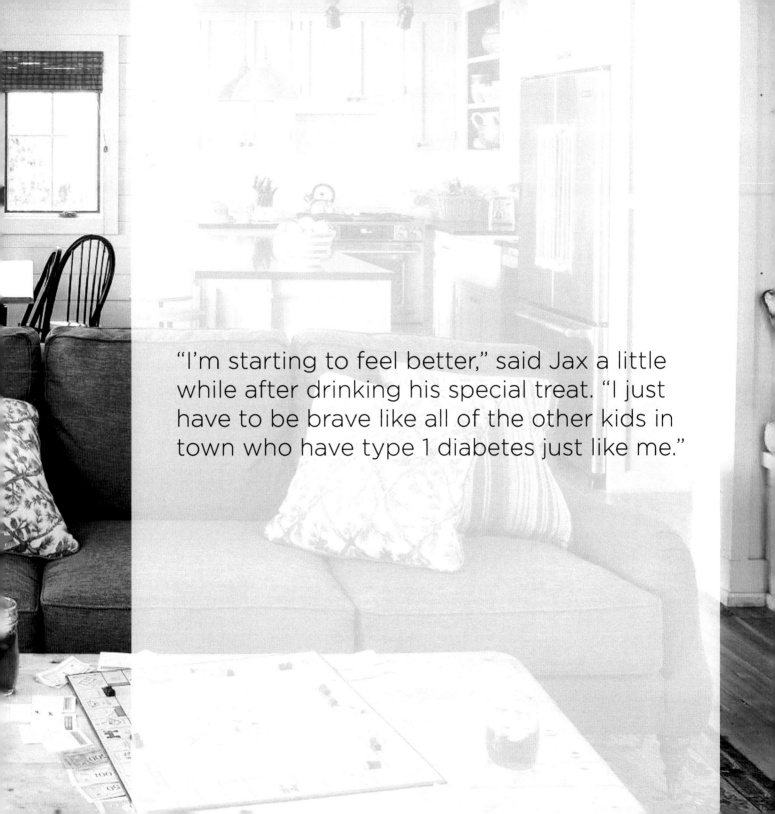

"I'm starting to feel better," said Jax a little while after drinking his special treat. "I just have to be brave like all of the other kids in town who have type 1 diabetes just like me."

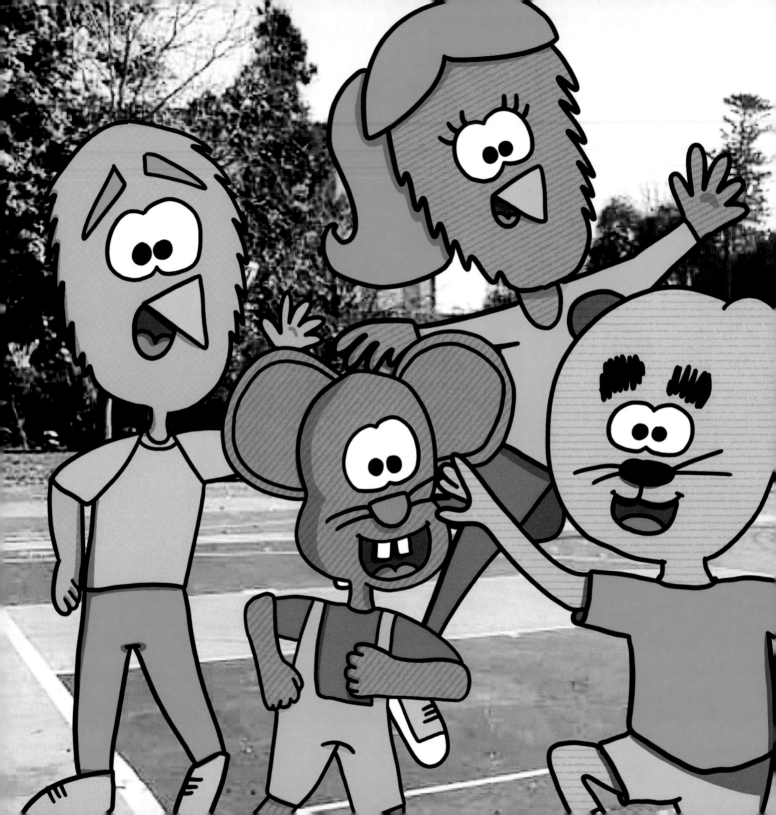

The End

Made in the USA
Columbia, SC
17 January 2021

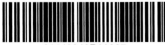

31149948R00027